46 Arthritis Preventing and Pain Relieving Juice Recipes:

The All-natural remedy to Controlling Your Arthritis Conditions Fast

By

Joe Correa CSN

COPYRIGHT

This publication is designed to provide accurate and authoritative information in regard to the subject matter covered. It is sold with the understanding that neither the author nor the publisher is engaged in rendering medical advice. If medical advice or assistance is needed, consult with a doctor. This book is considered a guide and should not be used in any way detrimental to your health. Consult with a physician before starting this nutritional plan to make sure it's right for you.

ACKNOWLEDGEMENTS

This book is dedicated to my friends and family that have had mild or serious illnesses so that you may find a solution and make the necessary changes in your life.

46 Arthritis Preventing and Pain Relieving Juice Recipes:

The All-natural remedy to Controlling Your Arthritis Conditions Fast

By

Joe Correa CSN

CONTENTS

ABOUT THE AUTHOR

After years of Research, I honestly believe in the positive effects that proper nutrition can have over the body and mind. My knowledge and experience has helped me live healthier throughout the years and which I have shared with family and friends. The more you know about eating and drinking healthier, the sooner you will want to change your life and eating habits.

Nutrition is a key part in the process of being healthy and living longer so get started today. The first step is the most important and the most significant.

INTRODUCTION

46 Arthritis Preventing and Pain Relieving Juice Recipes: The All-natural remedy to Controlling Your Arthritis Conditions Fast

By Joe Correa CSN

Arthritis is an autoimmune disease in which the joints are symmetrically affected by the inflammation, causing the pain and stiffness. There are about 100 different types of arthritis, but the most common ones are rheumatoid arthritis and osteoarthritis. Unlike rheumatoid arthritis which is an autoimmune disorder, osteoarthritis is described as a degenerative joint disease. The exact cause of arthritis is unknown, but there are many different factors that may affect the autoimmune response, including genetic susceptibility. Early symptoms for both types include painful swelling of joints, morning stiffness, and inflammation.

A proper nutrition plays an important role in reducing the risk of arthritis. Our modern diet, based on animal-derived foods, refined sugar, and foods that provoke the immune system response increases the sensitivity for inflammation which leads to this painful disease. With a good nutrition, consistency, and good lifestyle choices, your health will improve significantly and your body will get a chance to resist the inflammation. Furthermore, healthy, fresh, and unprocessed foods will reduce the risk of obesity which not only contributes to the onset and progress of arthritis but also makes your joints carry more weight. Excess weight directly damages your joints and contributes to both - development and progress of this disease.

The main reason I have created this great collection of arthritis preventing juice recipes was to give you a quick and simple way to get all the nutrients you need in order to boost your immune system, cleanse your body, and lose some weight all at the same time. Juicing is one of the best ways to nourish your body with amazingly valuable antioxidants and other important substances in just a few minutes. This collection of juices is especially practical for people with busy schedules who have very little to prepare everything. It's also a perfect option for those of you who don't enjoy eating specific fruits or vegetables throughout the day, but still want to get huge amounts of vitamins and minerals into their body.

I hope these powerful juice recipes will serve as a guide for your arthritis problems. These juices will make your digestion easier and will help eliminate dangerous toxins that lead to inflammation and arthritis. This book is all about getting the right nutrients you need in a more convenient way and preventing arthritis once and for all.

46 ARTHRITIS PREVENTING AND PAIN RELIEVING JUICE RECIPES: THE ALL-NATURAL REMEDY TO CONTROLLING YOUR ARTHRITIS CONDITIONS FAST

1.   Cherry Cucumber Juice

Ingredients:

2 cups of fresh cherries, pitted

1 large cucumber, sliced

1 large lemon, peeled

1 medium-sized Granny smith apple, cored

2 oz of water

Preparation:

Using a colander, wash the cherries under cold running water. Cut in half and remove the pits. Set aside.

Wash the cucumber and cut into thick slices. Set aside.

Peel the lemon and cut lengthwise in half. Set aside.

Wash the apple and remove the core. Cut into bite-sized pieces and set aside.

Now, combine cherries, cucumber, lemon, and apple in a juicer and process until juiced. Transfer to serving glasses and stir in the water. Add few ice cubes before serving.

Enjoy!

Nutritional information per serving: Kcal: 296, Protein: 6.6g, Carbs: 88.4g, Fats: 1.4g

2.   Orange Apricot Juice

Ingredients:

2 large oranges, peeled

2 large apricots, pitted

1 cup of pomegranate seeds

1 cup of green grapes

1 large lemon, peeled

1 small ginger slice, peeled

Preparation:

Peel the oranges and divide into wedges. Set aside.

Wash the apricots and cut in half. Remove the pits and cut into small pieces. Set aside.

Cut the top of the pomegranate fruit using a sharp knife. Slice down to each of the white membranes inside of the fruit. Pop the seeds into a measuring cup and set aside.

Peel the lemon and cut lengthwise in half. Set aside.

Peel the ginger slice and set aside.

Now, combine oranges, apricots, pomegranate, lemon, and ginger in a juicer. Process until well juiced and transfer to serving glasses. Refrigerate for 20 minutes before serving.

Nutritional information per serving: Kcal: 294, Protein: 7.2g, Carbs: 88.9g, Fats: 2.3g

3.   Blueberry Mint Juice

Ingredients:

1 cup of blueberries

1 cup of fresh mint, torn

1 large red apple, cored

1 large cucumber, sliced

2 oz of coconut water

Preparation:

Place the blueberries in a colander and wash under cold running water. Drain and set aside.

Wash the mint thoroughly and torn with hands. Set aside.

Wash the apple and cut in half. Remove the core and cut into bite-sized pieces. Set aside.

Wash the cucumber and gently peel it. Cut into thin slices and set aside.

Now, combine blueberries, mint, apple, and cucumber in a juicer. Process until juiced and transfer to serving glasses. Stir in the coconut water and refrigerate for 15 minutes, or add some ice before serving.

Enjoy!

Nutritional information per serving: Kcal: 258, Protein: 4.7g, Carbs: 74.6g, Fats: 1.6g

4. Strawberry Mango Juice

Ingredients:

6 large strawberries, chopped

1 cup of mango, peeled and chopped

1 cup of cantaloupe, chopped

1 large cucumber, sliced

2 oz of coconut water

Preparation:

Wash the strawberries and cut into bite-sized pieces. Set aside.

Peel the mango and cut into small chunks. Fill the measuring cup and reserve the rest for later.

Cut the cantaloupe in half and scoop out the seeds. Cut two wedges and peel them. Chop into chunks and fill the measuring cup. Reserve the rest of the cantaloupe in a refrigerator.

Wash the cucumber and cut into thick slices. Set aside.

Now, combine strawberries, mango, cantaloupe, and cucumber in a juicer and process until juiced. Transfer to serving glasses and stir in the coconut water. refrigerate for 30 minutes before serving.

Enjoy!

Nutritional information per serving: Kcal: 209, Protein: 5.3g, Carbs: 56.6g, Fats: 1.5g

5.   Avocado Citrus Juice

Ingredients:

1 cup of avocado, pitted and chopped

1 large cucumber, sliced

1 large lemon, peeled

1 cup of fresh spinach, torn

1 large lime, peeled

1 small ginger knob, peeled

3 oz of water

Preparation:

Peel the avocado and cut in half. Remove the pit and chop into chunks. Set aside.

Wash the cucumber and cut into thick slices. Set aside.

Peel the lemon and lime. Cut lengthwise in half and set aside.

Wash the spinach thoroughly and torn with hands. Set aside.

Peel the ginger knob and set aside.

Now, combine avocado, cucumber, lemon, lime, spinach, and ginger in a juicer. Process until juiced and transfer to serving glasses. Stir in the water and refrigerate for 20 minutes before serving.

Enjoy!

Nutritional information per serving: Kcal: 269, Protein: 6.7g, Carbs: 35g, Fats: 22.6g

6.   Artichoke Turmeric Juice

Ingredients:

1 large artichoke, peeled and chopped

1 cup of Brussels sprouts, trimmed

1 large carrot, sliced

1 cup of fresh celery, chopped

1 cup of turnip greens, chopped

1 large green apple, cored

½ tsp of turmeric, ground

2 oz of water

Preparation:

Using a sharp knife, trim off the outer leaves of the artichoke. Cut into small pieces and set aside.

Trim off the outer leaves of the Brussels sprouts and wash them thoroughly. Cut in half and set aside.

Wash the carrot and cut into thin slices. Set aside.

Wash the celery and chop it into bite-sized pieces. Set aside.

Wash the apple and cut in half. Remove the core and cut into bite-sized pieces. Set aside.

Wash the turnip greens thoroughly and torn with hands. Set aside.

Now, combine artichoke, Brussels sprouts, carrot, celery, turnip greens, and apple in a juicer. Process until well juiced and transfer to serving glasses. Stir in the turmeric and water. Add some ice before serving.

Nutritional information per serving: Kcal: 205, Protein: 11.3g, Carbs: 66.7g, Fats: 1.4g

7.   Watermelon Orange Juice

Ingredients:

2 cups of watermelon, chopped

1 large orange, peeled

1 cup of raspberries

1 large kiwi, peeled

2 oz coconut water

Preparation:

Cut the watermelon lengthwise. For 2 cups, you will need about 2 large wedges. Peel and cut into chunks. Remove the seeds and set aside. Reserve the rest of the melon for some other juices. Set aside.

Peel the orange and divide into wedges. Set aside.

Wash the raspberries thoroughly under cold running water. Drain and set aside.

Peel the kiwi and cut lengthwise in half. Set aside.

Now, combine watermelon, orange, raspberries, and kiwi in a juicer. Process until juiced and transfer to serving glasses. Stir in the coconut water and refrigerate for 15 minutes before serving.

Nutritional information per serving: Kcal: 232, Protein: 5.8g, Carbs: 71.4g, Fats: 1.8g

8.   Salted Beet Tomato Juice

Ingredients:

2 cups of beets, trimmed

1 large Roma tomato, chopped

1 large cucumber, sliced

3 large radishes, trimmed

½ tsp of fresh rosemary, chopped

¼ tsp of sea salt

1 oz of water

Preparation:

Wash the beets and trim off the green parts. Cut into small pieces and set aside.

Wash the tomato and place it in a bowl. Cut into bite-sized pieces and reserve the tomato juice while cutting. Set aside.

Wash the cucumber and cut into thin slices. Set aside.

Wash the radishes and trim off the green ends. Cut in half and set aside.

Now, combine beets, tomato, cucumber, radishes, and rosemary in a juicer. Process until well juiced and transfer to serving glasses. Stir in the salt and water. refrigerate for 10 minutes before serving.

Enjoy!

Nutritional information per serving: Kcal: 152, Protein: 8.2g, Carbs: 44.9g, Fats: 1.2g

9.   Pepper Squash Juice

Ingredients:

3 large red bell peppers, chopped

1 cup of butternut squash, cubed

1 cup of parsnip, sliced

1 tbsp of fresh parsley, chopped

2 oz of water

Preparation:

Wash the red bell peppers and cut lengthwise in half. Remove the seeds and chop into small pieces.

Peel the butternut squash and remove the seeds using a spoon. Cut into small cubes and fill the measuring cup. Reserve the rest of the squash for some other recipe. Wrap in a plastic foil and refrigerate.

Wash the parsnip and peel it. Cut into thin slices and set aside.

Now, combine bell peppers, butternut squash, parsnip, and parsley in a juicer. Process until well juiced and transfer to serving glasses. Stir in the water and add some ice.

Serve immediately.

Nutritional information per serving: Kcal: 238, Protein: 7.9g, Carbs: 70.2g, Fats: 2.1g

10.   Papaya Pomegranate Juice

Ingredients:

1 large papaya, peeled and chopped

1 cup of pomegranate seeds

1 large green apple, cored

1 tbsp of fresh mint, chopped

2 oz of water

Preparation:

Peel the papaya and cut lengthwise in half. Scoop out the black seeds and flesh using a spoon. Cut into small chunks and set aside.

Cut the top of the pomegranate fruit using a sharp knife. Slice down to each of the white membranes inside of the fruit. Pop the seeds into a measuring cup and set aside.

Wash the apple and cut in half. Using a sharp knife, remove the core and cut into bite-sized pieces. Set aside.

Now, combine papaya, pomegranate, apple, and mint in a juicer. Process until well juiced and transfer to serving glasses. Stir in the water and refrigerate for 15 minutes before serving.

Nutritional information per serving: Kcal: 438, Protein: 6.1g, Carbs: 129g, Fats: 3.4g

11.   Plum Blackberry Juice

Ingredients:

5 large plums, pitted

2 cups of blackberries

1 large lemon, peeled

1 cup of black grapes

1 medium-sized Golden delicious apple, cored

2 oz of water

1 tsp of liquid honey

Preparation:

Wash the plums and cut in half. Remove the pits and cut in small pieces. Set aside.

Wash the blackberries thoroughly under cold running water. Drain and set aside.

Peel the lemon and cut lengthwise in half. Set aside.

Wash the black grapes and set aside.

Wash the apple and cut in half. Remove the core and cut into bite-sized pieces. Set aside.

Now, combine plums, blackberries, lemon, black grapes, and apple in a juicer. Process until well juiced and transfer to serving glasses. Stir in the honey and water. Add some ice and serve immediately.

Enjoy!

Nutritional information per serving: Kcal: 344, Protein: 8g, Carbs: 110g, Fats: 3.1g

12.   Pineapple Lime Juice

Ingredients:

1 cup of pineapple chunks

2 large limes, peeled

1 cup of guava, chopped

1 large cucumber, sliced

1 tbsp of fresh basil, chopped

2 oz of water

Preparation:

Cut the top of a pineapple and peel it using a sharp knife. Cut into small chunks and fill the measuring cup. Reserve the rest of the pineapple in a refrigerator.

Peel the limes and cut lengthwise in half. Set aside.

Wash the guava and cut into chunks. Fill the measuring cup and reserve the rest for some other recipe in a refrigerator.

Wash the cucumber and cut into thin slices. Set aside.

Now, combine pineapple, limes, guava, cucumber, and basil in a juicer. Process until well juiced and transfer to serving glasses. Stir in the water and refrigerate for 15 minutes before serving.

Nutritional information per serving: Kcal: 158, Protein: 4.7g, Carbs: 47.9g, Fats: 1.1g

13.   Cranberry Pear Juice

Ingredients:

1 cup of cranberries

1 large pear, cored

1 large green apple, cored

3 large strawberries, chopped

1 large orange, peeled

¼ tsp of nutmeg, ground

2 oz of coconut water

Preparation:

Wash the cranberries thoroughly under cold running water. Drain and set aside.

Wash the pear and cut lengthwise in half. Remove the core and cut into bite-sized pieces. Set aside.

Wash the apple and cut in half. Remove the core and cut into bite-sized pieces. Set aside.

Wash the strawberries thoroughly and chop into small pieces. Set aside.

Peel the orange and divide into wedges. Set aside.

Now, combine pear, apple, strawberries, orange, and nutmeg in a juicer. Process until well juiced and transfer to serving glasses. Stir in the water and refrigerate or add some ice before serving.

Nutritional information per serving: Kcal: 158, Protein: 4.7g, Carbs: 47.9g, Fats: 1.1g

14.   Carrot Orange Juice

Ingredients:

5 large carrots, peeled

1 large orange, peeled and wedged

1 large lemon, peeled

1 cup of Romaine lettuce, torn

1 large cucumber, sliced

¼ tsp of turmeric, ground

Preparation:

Peel and wash the carrots. Cut into thin slices and set aside.

Peel the orange and divide into wedges. Set aside.

Peel the lemon and cut lengthwise in half. Set aside.

Wash the lettuce thoroughly and torn with hands. Set aside.

Wash the cucumber and cut into thin slices. Set aside.

Now, combine carrots, orange, lemon, lettuce, and cucumber in a juicer. Process until well juiced and transfer to serving glasses. stir in the turmeric and add some ice before serving. Enjoy!

Nutritional information per serving: Kcal: 232, Protein: 8.2g, Carbs: 74g, Fats: 1.7g

15.   Asparagus Collard Greens Juice

Ingredients:

1 cup of asparagus, trimmed

1 cup of collard greens, torn

1 cup of watercress, torn

1 green bell pepper, chopped

1 large cucumber, sliced

2 oz of water

¼ tsp of salt

Preparation:

Wash the asparagus and trim off the woody ends. Cut into bite-sized pieces and fill the measuring cup. Reserve the rest for some other juice.

Combine collard greens and watercress in a colander. Wash thoroughly under cold running water and torn with hands. Set aside.

Wash the bell pepper and lengthwise in half. Remove the seeds and chop into small pieces. Set aside.

Wash the cucumber and cut into thin slices. Set aside.

Now, combine asparagus, collard greens, bell pepper, and cucumber in a juicer and process until well juiced. Transfer to serving glasses and stir in the salt and water. refrigerate for 15 minutes before serving.

Nutritional information per serving: Kcal: 86, Protein: 8.2g, Carbs: 26.1g, Fats: 1g

16.   Sweet Potato Green Smoothie

Ingredients:

1 cup of sweet potatoes, peeled

1 large fennel, chopped

1 cup of Swiss chard, torn

1 cup of red leaf lettuce, torn

1 cup of fresh spinach, torn

1 small cauliflower head, chopped

1 large lemon, peeled

Preparation:

Peel the sweet potato and cut into small chunks. Fill the measuring cup and reserve the rest for some other juice.

Wash the fennel bulb and trim off the wilted outer layers. Cut into small chunks and set aside.

Combine Swiss chard, red leaf lettuce, and spinach in a colander. Wash under cold running water and drain. Torn with hands and set aside.

Trim off the outer leaves of cauliflower. Wash it and cut into small pieces. Set aside.

Peel the lemon and cut lengthwise in half. Set aside.

Now, combine potato, fennel, Swiss chard, cauliflower, and lemon in a juicer and process until well juiced. Transfer to serving glasses and add some ice before serving.

Nutritional information per serving: Kcal: 218, Protein: 14.3g, Carbs: 67.7g, Fats: 1.9g

17.   Fennel Brussels Sprouts Juice

Ingredients:

1 medium-sized fennel bulb, chopped

1 cup of Brussels sprouts, halved

1 large yellow bell pepper, chopped

1 large cucumber, sliced

¼ tsp of salt

2 oz of water

Preparation:

Trimm off the fennel stalks and wilted outer layers. Cut into bite-sized pieces and set aside.

Trim off the outer leaves and wash the Brussels sprouts. Cut in half and set aside.

Wash the bell pepper and cut lengthwise in half. Remove the seeds and chop into small pieces. Set aside.

Wash the cucumber and cut into thin slices. Set aside.

Now, combine fennel, Brussels sprouts, bell peppers, and cucumber in a juicer. Process until well juiced and stir in the salt and water. Refrigerate for 10 minutes before serving.

Nutritional information per serving: Kcal: 151, Protein: 9.7g, Carbs: 47.6g, Fats: 1.4g

18.   Watermelon Peach Juice

Ingredients:

1 cup of watermelon, cubed

2 large peaches, pitted

1 large green apple, cored

5 fresh cherries, pitted

3 oz of coconut water

Preparation:

Cut the watermelon lengthwise. For one cup, you will need about one large wedge. Peel and cut into chunks. Remove the seeds and set aside. Reserve the rest of the melon for some other juices.

Wash the peaches and cut in half. Remove the pits and cut into bite-sized pieces. Set aside.

Wash the apple and cut in half. Remove the core and cut into bite-sized pieces. Set aside.

Wash the cherries and cut in half. Remove the pits and set aside.

Now, process watermelon, peaches, apple, and cherries in a juicer. Transfer to serving glasses and stir in the coconut water. Add some ice and serve immediately.

Nutritional information per serving: Kcal: 276, Protein: 5.4g, Carbs: 47.6g, Fats: 1.6g

19. Spinach Apple Juice

Ingredients:

1 cup of fresh spinach, torn

1 large red apple, cored

1 cup of wild asparagus, trimmed

1 cup of collard greens, torn

1 cup of mustard greens, torn

2 oz of water

Preparation:

Combine spinach, collard greens, and mustard greens in a large colander. Wash under cold running water and drain. Torn with hands and set aside.

Wash the apple and cut in half. Remove the core and cut into bite-sized pieces. Set aside.

Now, combine spinach, collard greens, mustard greens, and apple in a juicer and process until well juiced. Transfer to serving glasses and stir in the water. refrigerate for 15 minutes before serving.

Enjoy!

Nutritional information per serving: Kcal: 207, Protein: 16.1g, Carbs: 58.6g, Fats: 2.5g

20.   Plum Cabbage Juice

Ingredients:

5 large plums, pitted

1 cup of purple cabbage, chopped

1 cup of blackberries

1 large cucumber, sliced

2 oz of water

Preparation:

Wash the plums and cut in half. Remove the pits and cut into quarters. Set aside.

Wash the cabbage thoroughly under cold running water. Drain and roughly chop it. Set aside.

Wash the blackberries under cold running water using a colander. Slightly drain and set aside.

Wash the cucumber and cut into thin slices. Set aside.

Now, combine plums, cabbage, blackberries, and cucumber in a juicer and process until juice. Transfer to serving glasses and stir in the water. refrigerate for 15 minutes before serving.

Nutritional information per serving: Kcal: 221, Protein: 7.5g, Carbs: 69.1g, Fats: 2.1g

21.   Crookneck Squash Tomato Juice

Ingredients:

1 cup of crookneck squash, chopped

1 large tomato, chopped

1 large lemon, peeled

1 large orange, peeled

1 large pear, cored and chopped

2 oz of water

1 tsp of liquid honey

Preparation:

Wash the crookneck squash and cut in half. Scoop out the seeds using a spoon. Cut into small chunks and fill the measuring cup. Reserve the rest for another juice.

Wash the tomato and place it in a bowl. Cut into bite-sized pieces and reserve the juice while cutting. Set aside.

Peel the lemon and cut lengthwise in half. Set aside.

Peel the orange and divide into wedges. Set aside.

Wash the pear and cut lengthwise in half. Remove the core and cut into bite-sized pieces. Set aside.

Now, combine crookneck squash, tomato, lemon, orange, and pear in a juicer. Process until well juiced and transfer to serving glasses. Stir in the water and honey. Add some ice and serve immediately.

Nutritional information per serving: Kcal: 201, Protein: 5.9g, Carbs: 66.1g, Fats: 1.3g

22.   Cauliflower Leek Juice

Ingredients:

1 small cauliflower head, chopped

3 large leeks, chopped

1 large lime, peeled

1 large zucchini, chopped

2 oz of water

Preparation:

Trim off the outer leaves of cauliflower. Wash it and cut into small pieces. Set aside.

Wash the leeks and cut into small pieces. Set aside.

Peel the lime and cut lengthwise in half. Set aside.

Peel the zucchini and cut in half. Scrape out the seeds and cut into small chunks. Set aside.

Now, combine cauliflower, leeks, lime, and zucchini in a juicer. Process until well juiced and stir in the water. Refrigerate for 10 minutes before serving.

Enjoy!

Nutritional information per serving: Kcal: 241, Protein: 13.2g, Carbs: 64.7g, Fats: 2.6g

23.   Raspberry Beet Juice

Ingredients:

2 cups of raspberries

1 large green apple, cored

1 cup of beets, chopped

1 cup of fresh basil, torn

1 large lemon, peeled

3 oz of water

Preparation:

Wash the raspberries under cold running water using a colander. Drain and set aside.

Wash the apple and cut in half. Remove the core and cut into bite-sized pieces. Set aside.

Wash the beets and trim off the green ends. Cut into small pieces and fill the measuring cup. Reserve the greens for some other juice.

Wash the basil thoroughly under cold running water and torn with hands. Set aside.

Peel the lemon and cut lengthwise in half. Set aside.

Now, combine raspberries, apple, beets, basil, and lemon in a juicer. Process until well juiced. Stir in the water and refrigerate for 10 minutes before serving.

Enjoy!

Nutritional information per serving: Kcal: 218, Protein: 7.5g, Carbs: 76.4g, Fats: 2.5g

24.   Apricot Pomegranate Juice

Ingredients:

1 large apricot, pitted

1 cup of pomegranate seeds

1 large lemon, peeled

1 large orange, wedged

1 large carrot, peeled

2 oz of coconut water

Preparation:

Wash the apricot and cut in half. Remove the pit and cut into small pieces. Set aside.

Cut the top of the pomegranate fruit using a sharp knife. Slice down to each of the white membranes inside of the fruit. Pop the seeds into measuring cup and set aside.

Peel the lemon and cut lengthwise in half. Set aside.

Peel the orange and divide into wedges. Set aside.

Peel and wash the carrot. Cut into thin slices and set aside.

Now, combine apricot, pomegranate seeds, lemon, orange, and carrot in a juicer. Process until well juiced and transfer to serving glasses. Stir in the coconut water and add few ice cubes before serving.

Nutritional information per serving: Kcal: 241, Protein: 7.3g, Carbs: 73.9g, Fats: 2.3g

25.   Broccoli Kale Juice

Ingredients:

2 cups of broccoli, trimmed

1 cup of fresh kale, torn

1 cup of fresh parsley, torn

1 large green apple, chopped

1 cup of fresh spinach, torn

2 oz of water

Preparation:

Wash the broccoli under cold running water and cut into small pieces. Set aside.

Combine parsley, kale, and spinach in a colander and wash under cold running water. Drain and torn with hands. Set aside.

Wash the apple and cut in half. Remove the core and cut into bite-sized pieces. Set aside.

Now, combine broccoli, kale, parsley, apple, and spinach in a juicer. Process until well juiced and stir in the water.

Refrigerate for 20 minutes before serving.

Nutritional information per serving: Kcal: 223, Protein: 20.4g, Carbs: 62.1g, Fats: 3.5g

26. Mango Cherry Juice

Ingredients:

1 cup of mango, chopped

1 cup of fresh cherries, pitted

2 cup of green grapes

1 large lemon, peeled

2 oz of water

Preparation:

Wash the mango and cut into chunks. Fill the measuring cup and reserve the rest for some other juice. Set aside.

Wash the cherries and cut in half. Remove the pits and set aside.

Wash the grapes and fill the measuring cup. Reserve the rest for some other juice. Set aside.

Peel the lemon and cut lengthwise in half. Set aside.

Now, combine mango, cherries, grapes, and lemon in a juicer and process until well juiced. Transfer to serving glasses and stir in the water.

Add few ice cubes and serve immediately.

Nutritional information per serving: Kcal: 302, Protein: 4.8g, Carbs: 86.3g, Fats: 1.7g

27.   Grapefruit Apple Juice

Ingredients:

2 large grapefruits, peeled

1 large red apple, cored

2 large strawberries, chopped

1 small ginger knob, peeled

2 oz of coconut water

Preparation:

Peel the grapefruits and divide into wedges. Set aside.

Wash the apple and cut in half. Remove the core and cut into bite-sized pieces. Set aside.

Wash the strawberries and cut into small pieces. Set aside.

Peel the ginger knob and set aside.

Now, combine grapefruits, apple, strawberries, and ginger in a juicer. Process until well juiced and transfer to serving glasses. Stir in the coconut water and refrigerate for 15 minutes, or add some ice before serving.

Nutritional information per serving: Kcal: 302, Protein: 4.8g, Carbs: 86.3g, Fats: 1.7g

28.   Pumpkin Nutmeg Juice

Ingredients:

2 cups of pumpkin, cubed

1 large green apple, cored

1 large cucumber, sliced

1 cup of Swiss chard, torn

2 oz of water

¼ tsp of nutmeg, ground

Preparation:

Peel the pumpkin and cut in half. Scoop out the seeds using a spoon. Cut one large wedge and peel it. Cut into small cubes and fill the measuring cup. Reserve the rest for some other juice.

Wash the apple and cut in half. Remove the core and cut into bite-sized pieces. Set aside.

Wash the cucumber and cut into thin slices. Set aside.

Wash the Swiss chard thoroughly under cold running water. Drain and torn with hands. Set aside.

Now, combine pumpkin, apple, cucumber, and Swiss chards in a juicer. Process until well juiced and stir in the water and nutmeg. Refrigerate for 15 minutes before serving.

Nutritional information per serving: Kcal: 196, Protein: 5.8g, Carbs: 55.4g, Fats: 1.1g

29.   Celery Green Bean Juice

Ingredients:

2 cups of celery, chopped

1 cup of green beans, chopped

1 cup of fresh mint, torn

1 cup of beet greens, torn

1 large cucumber, sliced

2 oz of water

¼ tsp of salt

Preparation:

Wash the celery and cut into small pieces. Set aside.

Wash the green beans and cut into bite-sized pieces. Set aside.

Combine mint and beet greens in a colander. Wash under cold running water and torn with hands. Set aside.

Wash the cucumber and cut into thin slices. Set aside.

Now, combine celery, green beans, mint, beet greens, and cucumber in a juicer. Process until well juiced and transfer to serving glasses. Stir in the water and salt.

Refrigerate for 10 minutes before serving.

Nutritional information per serving: Kcal: 91, Protein: 6.1g, Carbs: 26.1g, Fats: 1g

30.   Strawberry Peach Juice

Ingredients:

1 cup of strawberries, chopped

2 large peaches, pitted

1 large green apple, cored

1 large lemon, peeled

1 large kiwi, peeled

1 large orange, peeled

2 oz of water

Preparation:

Wash the strawberries under cold running water. Remove the green parts and cut into bite-sized pieces. Set aside.

Wash the peaches and cut in half. Remove the pits and cut into small pieces. Set aside.

Wash the apple and cut half. Remove the core and cut into bite-sized pieces. Set aside.

Peel the lemon and kiwi. Cut lengthwise in half and set aside.

Now, combine strawberries, peaches, apple, lemon, and kiwi in a juicer and process until well juiced. Transfer to serving glasses and stir in the water. Add some ice and serve immediately.

Enjoy!

Nutritional information per serving: Kcal: 345, Protein: 7.8g, Carbs: 105g, Fats: 2.3g

31.   Sour Pepper Lemon Juice

Ingredients:

1 large red bell pepper, chopped

1 large lemon, peeled

1 cup of beets, chopped

1 large cucumber, sliced

1 tsp of balsamic vinegar

¼ tsp of salt

2 oz of water

Preparation:

Wash the bell pepper and cut in half. Remove the seeds and chop into small pieces. Set aside.

Peel the lemon and cut lengthwise in half. Set aside.

Wash the beets and trim off the green ends. Cut into bite-sized pieces and fill the measuring cup. Reserve the rest for some other juice. Set aside.

Wash the cucumber and cut into thin slices. Set aside.

Now, combine bell pepper, lemon, beets, and cucumber in a juicer. Process until well juiced and transfer to serving glasses. Stir in the balsamic vinegar, salt, and water.

Refrigerate for 20 minutes before serving.

Nutritional information per serving: Kcal: 130, Protein: 6.4g, Carbs: 39.2g, Fats: 1.2g

32.   Blackberry Apricot Juice

Ingredients:

1 cup of blackberries

1 cup of raspberries

3 large apricots, pitted

1 large red apple, cored

3 large carrots, peeled

Preparation:

Combine blackberries and raspberries in a colander. Wash under cold running water and slightly drain. Set aside.

Wash the apricots and cut in half. Remove the pits and cut into bite-sized pieces. Set aside.

Wash the apple and cut in half. Remove the core and cut into small pieces.

Wash and peel the carrots. Cut into thin slices and set aside.

Now, combine blackberries, raspberries, apricots, apple, and carrots in a juicer. Process until well juiced and transfer to serving glasses. Stir in the water and refrigerate for 20 minutes before serving.

Enjoy!

Nutritional information per serving: Kcal: 301, Protein: 7.6g, Carbs: 97.4g, Fats: 2.9g

33.   Strawberry Avocado Juice

Ingredients:

5 large strawberries, chopped

1 cup of avocado, pitted

1 cup of fresh mint, chopped

1 large apple, cored

1 large lemon, peeled

1 large cucumber, sliced

Preparation:

Wash the strawberries and cut into small pieces. Set aside.

Peel the avocado and cut lengthwise in half. Remove the pit and cut into chunks and fill the measuring cup. Reserve the rest for later.

Wash the mint thoroughly and torn with hands. Set aside.

Wash the apple and cut in half. Remove the core and cut into bite-sized pieces. Set aside.

Peel the lemon and cut lengthwise in half. Set aside.

Wash the cucumber and cut into thin slices. Set aside.

Now, combine strawberries, avocado, mint, lemon, and cucumber in a juicer and process until juiced. Transfer to serving glasses and stir in the water. Add some ice and serve immediately.

Nutritional information per serving: Kcal: 376, Protein: 8.1g, Carbs: 67.8g, Fats: 23.3g

34.   Cantaloupe Carrot Juice

Ingredients:

1 cup of cantaloupe, cubed

3 large carrots, sliced

1 large orange, peeled

1 large green apple, cored

2 oz of coconut water

Preparation:

Cut the cantaloupe in half. Scoop out the seeds and flesh. Cut two wedges and peel them. Chop into cubes and set aside. Reserve the rest of the cantaloupe in a refrigerator.

Wash and peel the carrots. Cut into thin slices and set aside.

Peel the orange and divide into wedges. Set aside.

Wash the apple and cut in half. Remove the core and cut into bite-sized pieces. Set aside.

Now, combine cantaloupe, carrots, orange, and apple in a juicer. Process until well juiced and stir in the coconut water.

Nutritional information per serving: Kcal: 277, Protein: 6g, Carbs: 83g, Fats: 1.4g

35.   Pomegranate Pepper Juice

Ingredients:

1 cup of pomegranate seeds

1 large red bell pepper, chopped

1 cup of cranberries

4 large plums, pitted

1 large green apple, cored

Preparation:

Cut the top of the pomegranate fruit using a sharp knife. Slice down to each of the white membranes inside of the fruit. Pop the seeds into a measuring cup and set aside.

Wash the bell pepper and cut lengthwise in half. Remove the seeds and cut into small pieces. Set aside.

Wash the cranberries thoroughly and drain. Set aside.

Wash the plums and cut in half. Remove the pits and cut into bite-sized pieces. Set aside.

Wash the apple and cut in half. Remove the core and cut into bite-sized pieces. Set aside.

Now, combine pomegranate, cranberries, plums, and apple in a juicer. Process until well juiced and add some ice before serving.

Enjoy!

Nutritional information per serving: Kcal: 277, Protein: 6g, Carbs: 83g, Fats: 1.4g

36.   Zucchini Kiwi Juice

Ingredients:

1 large zucchini, seeded

3 large kiwis, peeled

1 large lime, peeled

1 cup of pomegranate seeds

1 large orange, peeled

Preparation:

Wash the zucchini and cut in half. Scoop out the seeds using a spoon. Cut into small chunks and set aside.

Peel the kiwis and lime. Cut lengthwise in half and set aside.

Cut the top of the pomegranate fruit using a sharp knife. Slice down to each of the white membranes inside of the fruit. Pop the seeds into a measuring cup and set aside.

Peel the orange and divide into wedges. Set aside.

Now, process kiwis, zucchini, lime, pomegranate seeds, and orange in a juicer.

Transfer to a serving glasses and add some ice cubes before serving.

Nutritional information per serving: Kcal: 183, Protein: 8.5g, Carbs: 52.6g, Fats: 1.6g

37.   Blueberry Mango Juice

Ingredients:

1 cup of mango, chopped

1 cup of blueberries

1 large cucumber, sliced

1 large green apple, cored

2 oz of water

Preparation:

Wash the mango and cut into chunks. Fill the measuring cup and reserve the rest for some other juice. Set aside.

Place the blueberries in a colander and wash under cold running water. Drain and set aside.

Wash the apple and remove the core. Cut into bite-sized pieces and set aside.

Now, combine mango, blueberries, and apple in a juicer and process until juiced.

Transfer to serving glasses and stir in the water. Add some ice before serving and enjoy!

Nutritional information per serving: Kcal: 180, Protein: 5.9g, Carbs: 63.5g, Fats: 1.1g

38.   Carrot Lemon Juice

Ingredients:

5 large carrots, sliced

2 large lemons, peeled

1 large green apple, cored

1 cup of Romaine lettuce

2 oz of water

Preparation:

Wash the carrots and cut into thick slices. Set aside.

Peel the lemons and cut lengthwise in half. Set aside.

Wash the apple and remove the core. Cut into bite-sized pieces and set aside.

Wash the lettuce thoroughly under cold running water. Torn with hands and set aside.

Now, process carrots, lettuce, lemon, and apple in a juicer. Transfer to serving glasses and add some ice before serving.

Enjoy!

Nutritional information per serving: Kcal: 232, Protein: 6.1g, Carbs: 74.9g, Fats: 1.7g

39.   Guava Lime Juice

Ingredients:

1 large guava, peeled

1 large lime, peeled

2 large oranges, peeled

1 large cucumber, sliced

2 oz of water

Preparation:

Peel and wash the guava. Cut into small chunks and set aside.

Peel the lime and cut lengthwise in half. Set aside.

Peel the oranges and divide into wedges. Set aside.

Wash the cucumber and cut into thin slices. Set aside.

Now, combine lime, guava, orange, and cucumber in a juicer and process until juiced.

Transfer to serving glasses and stir in the water. Add some ice and serve immediately.

Nutritional information per serving: Kcal: 210, Protein: 7g, Carbs: 65.7g, Fats: 1.3g

40. Celery Lemon Juice

Ingredients:

1 large lemon, peeled

1 cup of celery, chopped

1 cup of fresh mint, chopped

1 cup of fresh spinach, chopped

2 oz of water

Preparation:

Peel the lemon and cut lengthwise in half. Set aside.

Wash the celery stalks and chop into small pieces. Fill the measuring cup and set aside.

Wash the spinach and mint in a colander. Chop and place in a medium bowl. Set aside.

Now, combine lemon, celery, mint, and spinach in a juicer and process until juiced. Transfer to serving glasses and stir in the water.

Refrigerate for 10 minutes before serving.

Nutritional information per serving: Kcal: 35, Protein: 3.1g, Carbs: 13.2g, Fats: 0.7g

41. Basil Lemon Juice

Ingredients:

1 cup of fresh basil, chopped

1 large lemon, peeled

1 cup of Swiss chard, chopped

1 large green apple, cored

1 cup of fresh mint, chopped

2 oz of water

Preparation:

Combine basil, Swiss chard, and mint in a large colander. Wash thoroughly under cold running water. Chop into small pieces and set aside.

Peel the lemon and cut lengthwise in half.

Wash the apple and cut in half. Remove the core and cut into bite-sized pieces. Set aside.

Now, combine basil, Swiss chard, mint, lemon, and apple in a juicer and process until well juiced. Transfer to serving glasses and stir in the water.

Refrigerate for 10 minutes before serving.

Enjoy!

Nutritional information per serving: Kcal: 126, Protein: 3.9g, Carbs: 39.1g, Fats: 1.1g

42.　　Pineapple Carrot Juice

Ingredients:

1 cup of pineapple chunks

2 large carrots, sliced

1 cup of watercress, torn

1 large lime, peeled

1 small ginger knob, peeled

2 oz of water

Preparation:

Peel the pineapple and cut into small chunks. Set aside.

Wash and peel the carrots. Cut into thin slices and set aside.

Wash the watercress thoroughly under cold running water. Torn with hands and set aside.

Peel the lime and cut lengthwise in half. Set aside.

Peel the ginger root knob and cut into small pieces. Set aside.

Now, combine pineapple, carrots, watercress, lemon, and ginger in a juicer and process until well juiced.

Transfer to serving glasses and stir in water.

Add some ice and serve.

Nutritional information per serving: Kcal: 135, Protein: 3.3g, Carbs: 40.6g, Fats: 3.3g

43.   Orange Apple Juice

Ingredients:

3 large oranges, peeled

1 large green apple, cored

1 cup of fresh asparagus, trimmed

¼ tsp of turmeric, ground

2 oz of water

Preparation:

Peel the oranges and divide into wedges. Set aside.

Wash the apple and remove the core. Cut into bite-sized pieces and set aside.

Wash the asparagus thoroughly under cold running water and trim off the woody ends. Cut into small pieces and set aside.

Now, combine oranges, apple, and asparagus in a juicer and process until juiced. Transfer to serving glasses and stir in the turmeric and water.

Refrigerate for 10 minutes before serving.

Nutritional information per serving: Kcal: 316, Protein: 9.1g, Carbs: 98.1g, Fats: 1.2g

44.   Grapefruit Kiwi Juice

Ingredients:

2 large grapefruits, peeled

1 large kiwi, peeled

1 large lime, peeled

2 large celery stalks, chopped

1 cup of red leaf lettuce, chopped

2 oz of water

Preparation:

Peel the grapefruit and divide into wedges. Set aside.

Peel the kiwi and lime. Cut in half and set aside.

Wash and chop the celery stalks into small pieces. Set aside.

Wash the lettuce thoroughly under cold running water and roughly chop it. Set aside.

Now, combine grapefruit, kiwi, celery, and lettuce in a juicer and process until well juiced.

Transfer to serving glasses and stir in the water. Serve immediately.

Nutritional information per serving: Kcal: 233, Protein: 6g, Carbs: 70.7g, Fats: 1.3g

45.   Beet Pear Juice

Ingredients:

2 cups of beets, chopped

1 large pear, cored

1 large red bell pepper, chopped

1 large lemon, peeled

1 small ginger root slice, peeled

3 oz of water

Preparation:

Wash the beets and trim off the green ends. Cut into small pieces and fill the measuring cup. Reserve the greens for some other juice. Set aside.

Wash the pear and cut in half. Remove the core and cut into bite-sized pieces. Set aside.

Wash the bell pepper and cut in half. Remove the seeds and cut into small pieces. Set aside.

Peel the lemon and cut lengthwise in half. Set aside.

Peel the ginger slice and cut in half. Set aside.

Now, combine beets, pear, bell pepper, lemon, and ginger in a juicer. Process until well juiced and transfer to serving glasses.

Stir in the water and add some ice before serving.

Enjoy!

Nutritional information per serving: Kcal: 239, Protein: 7.5g, Carbs: 76.7g, Fats: 1.4g

46.   Leek Kale Juice

Ingredients:

3 large leeks, chopped

1 cup of fresh kale, chopped

1 cup of broccoli, chopped

1 large cucumber, sliced

1 garlic clove, peeled

1 tsp of fresh rosemary, chopped

2 oz of water

Preparation:

Wash the leeks and cut into bite-sized pieces. Set aside.

Wash the kale thoroughly under cold running water and chop into small pieces. Set aside.

Wash the broccoli and cut into small pieces. Fill the measuring cup and reserve the rest for some other juice. Set aside.

Wash the cucumber and cut into thin slices. Set aside.

Peel the garlic clove and cut in half. Set aside.

Now, combine leeks, kale, broccoli, cucumber, and garlic in a juicer. Process until well juiced.

Transfer to serving glasses and stir in the water. You can add a pinch of salt, but this is optional.

Serve immediately.

Nutritional information per serving: Kcal: 231, Protein: 11.6g, Carbs: 61.6g, Fats: 2.1g

ADDITIONAL TITLES FROM THIS AUTHOR

70 Effective Meal Recipes to Prevent and Solve Being Overweight: Burn Fat Fast by Using Proper Dieting and Smart Nutrition

By Joe Correa CSN

48 Acne Solving Meal Recipes: The Fast and Natural Path to Fixing Your Acne Problems in Less Than 10 Days!

By Joe Correa CSN

41 Alzheimer's Preventing Meal Recipes: Reduce or Eliminate Your Alzheimer's Condition in 30 Days or Less!

By Joe Correa CSN

70 Effective Breast Cancer Meal Recipes: Prevent and Fight Breast Cancer with Smart Nutrition and Powerful Foods

By Joe Correa CSN

www.ingramcontent.com/pod-product-compliance
Lightning Source LLC
Chambersburg PA
CBHW051031030426
42336CB00015B/2823